A SUMMARY, REVIEW &
ANALYSIS OF

DR. DAVID PERLMUTTER'S

GRAIN BRAIN

By

SAVE TIME SUMMARIES

Note to Readers: We encourage you to first order a copy of Dr. David Perlmutter's full book, _Grain Brain: The Surprising Truth about Wheat, Carbs, and Sugar--Your Brain's Silent Killers_ before you read this unofficial Book Summary & Review. Most readers use this guide by first reading a chapter from the full copy, and then reading the corresponding section from this Book Summary & Review. Others prefer to read the entire book from cover-to-cover, and then review using this review and analysis.

Other Amazon Kindle Ebooks from *Save Time Summaries:*

Summary of Robert Lustig's _Fat Chance -- Battling Sugar, Obesity & Disease_

Summary of Stephen Covey's _The 7 Habits of Highly Effective People_

TABLE OF CONTENTS

Dr. David Perlmutter believes that gluten is the source of all evil in the human body, and he offers his readers science, case histories, and medical studies to support his claims. In his medical practice, Dr. Perlmutter routinely tests patients for gluten sensitivity, as he believes that condition affects all areas of the body, not only a patient's digestive organs. In *Grain Brain*, Perlmutter makes the case that gluten in particular, and carbohydrates in general, are slowly killing your brain and will eventually lead to, at the minimum, impaired memory and cognitive abilities, and at the maximum, Alzheimer's disease and early death.

After making his case for the danger lurking in your breakfast bagel, Perlmutter outlines the lifestyle changes that will ensure optimum health: a diet rich in healthy fats and low in carbs, increased aerobic exercise, and good sleep habits. He also offers his readers a list of foods that support his recommendations, menu plans, and recipes that promise great taste and a sated appetite.

What Perlmutter does not offer his readers are any studies that refute his claims, though there are many of them to be found with a simple Internet search, including doctors and scientists responding directly to Perlmutter's theories. There are a number of other points he avoids in his quest to break his reader of the carb habit.

Perlmutter writes extensively of humankind's Paleolithic ancestors and the ideal hunter-gatherer diet. He proposes that these early people ate diets almost entirely consisting of fat, with the occasional seasonal berries and plants, and focuses on their freedom from Alzheimer's disease or dementia as proof that this diet is the optimum choice for human health. This opens up questions Perlmutter doesn't address, but that leap to the reader's mind. One, how does Perlmutter, or anyone, know what people ate 10,000 years ago? A more logical assumption would be they existed on a diet high in plant-based food, since that would have been easier to obtain than trapping or hunting animals using primitive weapons. Two, how likely is it Paleolithic humans would have lived long enough to contract Alzheimer's or dementia, as average lifespan was in the 30-year range? Three, how does Perlmutter know they didn't suffer from degenerative neurological disease? There are no medical records from 10,000 years ago.

Another fact Perlmutter ignores is the significant drop in weight and heart disease following World War II. Americans' improved health was contributed to the rationing of meat and dairy products during and after the war. He also ignores the hundreds, if not thousands, of years during which humans took a significant portion of their calories from carbohydrates, including grain, and the many areas of the world where they continue to do so. Even in modern times, when neurological disorders run rampant in America, the same issues are not found in places with carbohydrate-rich diets. As is typical in best-selling diet books, Perlmutter posits that there is a single, simple solution to neurological health. In reality, there are likely a host of contributing factors to the rise in diagnoses of dementia, Alzheimer's, and other mental and behavioral disorders.

Dr. Perlmutter does state his theories compellingly, and the reader will likely decide to begin a four-week plan immediately upon finishing reading. He writes well, with an engaging and knowledgeable style. If nothing else, his readers will likely incorporate some healthful lifestyle changes after reading his book, and that's a good thing in today's society.

Summary

Diseases that eventually lead to death are often chronic, the symptoms and complications accumulating over time until the body gives out. This is especially true in diseases of the brain, such as Alzheimer's disease. Alzheimer's and other forms of dementia obstruct the mind's ability to reason and remember, and people fear it more than they fear cancer or even death.

Common perceptions about Alzheimer's include the ideas that it's genetic or an unavoidable part of old age. Degenerative diseases of the brain are not inevitable. Rather, their cause can be found in the human diet, specifically in grains, not only the refined grains found in white bread and pasta, but in all grains: whole wheat, live grain, etc. "I am calling what is arguably our most beloved dietary staple a terrorist group that bullies our most precious organ, the brain." Grains are not the only culprit; all carbohydrates are detrimental to the brain's health. The information presented in *Grain Brain* is based on evolution and scientific fact and demonstrates not only the cause of brain disease, but also how to prevent it.

It is well documented that overall health can be improved through healthy habits. Due to the misconception that diseases of the brain are genetic or inevitable, brain health has not been viewed through this same preventative care lens.

During the last century, the shift to a low-fat, high-carb diet has led directly to modern ailments such as depression, chronic headaches, and attention deficit disorder. America's costliest ailments are diabetes and brain disease. Diabetes also doubles one's risk for Alzheimer's. Genetics also plays a significant role in how people process and respond to food. Modern grain is substantially altered from the wheat consumed by our ancient hunter-gatherer ancestors. Humans are not genetically equipped for the modern diet.

The modern approach to health is illness-centered, with patients looking to doctors for pills instead of focusing on wellness. Those prescriptions often result in dangerous side effects. *Grain Brain* offers a health-oriented approach, one that will inspire the reader to make immediate lifestyle changes.

Key Take-Aways

- Diseases of the brain are preventable.

- The food you eat may be slowly killing your brain.

Summary

People tend to consider brain dysfunction to be a whim of chance. The reality is that brain disease is the result of habits over time, thus it is preventable. A short true/false questionnaire gauges a person's risk factors and reveals neurological problems currently manifesting in the form of headaches, sexual dysfunction, and seizures (among other troubles). It also signals the likelihood of future mental decline.

A single "true" answer increases one's risk of neurological disorder; the risk rises as the number of "true" answers rise. Though neurological illness can't be cured, it can be prevented. Additionally, there are a number of medical tests that may help determine neurological health.

1. Fasting blood glucose: measures the amount of sugar in one's blood

2. Hemoglobin A1C: determines average blood sugar levels over a 90-day period

3. Fructosamine: measures average blood sugar over two to three weeks

4. Fasting insulin: measures insulin levels, which rise earlier than sugar levels. It is therefore an early indicator of diabetes risk

5. Homocysteine: higher levels of this amino acid indicate risk of a number of heart and brain diseases

6. Vitamin D: a critical brain hormone

7. C-reactive protein (CRP): indicates inflammation

8. Cyrex array 3: tests gluten sensitivity

9. Cyrex array 4: measures sensitivities more likely in people with a gluten intolerance

Key Take-Aways

- Cognizance of personal habits that increase one's risk of brain disease is vital to preventing it.

- A number of medical tests are available to gauge risk as well.

CHAPTER 1

Summary

Preventable, non-communicable disease accounts for more worldwide deaths than all other diseases combined. Though the average lifespan has increased dramatically in recent decades, this is due to decreases in infant mortality. In their later years, humans haven't had the same success in preventing and combating disease.

The cause of brain disease is largely dietary. Diet is not the sole cause of brain disorders, but many of these diseases are often the result of overconsumption of carbohydrates and under-representation of healthy fats in the diet. This is evident when Alzheimer's is considered alongside diet-induced diabetes.

Humans' ancient hunter-gatherer ancestors had brains very similar to the modern human. For survival, the human brain evolved to seek a diet high in both sugars and fats. Hunter-gatherers, after much effort, would have found only fats from animal protein and sugars found naturally in plants. In the modern age, humans find food easily, but it is in the form of processed fats and sugars. This difference affects how we age and determines our susceptibility to neurological disorders.

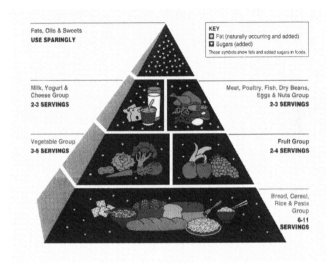

(Photo courtesy of Huffingtonpost.com)

The human body evolved to take glucose, the body's main source of energy, and store it for future use in times of scarcity. Additionally, it began to convert fats and proteins into glucose. Insulin, created by the pancreas, is the hormone that allows glucose to pass from blood cells to the body for use as energy. Healthy cells are easily affected by insulin, but cells with consistent exposure to the hormone aren't as receptive, so they don't absorb glucose. In response, the pancreas creates more insulin. If this cycle continues, high blood sugar and type 2 diabetes results. This toxicity has many effects, one of which is Alzheimer's.

Type 1 diabetes is a different disease. People with type 1 diabetes, approximately 5 percent of all diabetics, have a deficiency of insulin and must take daily injections of the hormone to balance their blood sugar. Type 2 diabetes is generally diagnosed in adulthood, whereas type 1 diabetics are typically diagnosed during childhood or adolescence. Type 1 cannot be cured, whereas type 2 may be cured through diet and exercise.

In 2005, it was proposed that Alzheimer's is a third type of diabetes. Further studies demonstrate the link between diet and Alzheimer's, opening the possibility of preventing the disease, as well as other brain disorders. Insulin resistance leads to the buildup of plaques found in the brains of Alzheimer's patients. Obese people and those with type 2 diabetes are at higher risk of developing Alzheimer's disease. An estimated 100 million people will be diagnosed with Alzheimer's disease by 2050. Type 2 diabetes cases have tripled over the past four decades.

What factors likely contribute to Alzheimer's?

1. Chronic high blood sugar levels

2. Consumption of too many carbohydrates

3. A low-fat diet

4. Undiagnosed gluten sensitivity

Gluten sensitivity is one of the highest threats to humanity's health. Neural dysfunction such as dementia, epilepsy, ADHD, and headaches may be caused by gluten, which up to 40 percent of people cannot process, and it is found in more than wheat-based products. Inflammation causes a number of degenerative conditions, and gluten causes inflammation of neural pathways, of which people are largely unaware. If gluten is bad, studies show that cholesterol and non-trans fat are good, as they reduce risk for brain disease.

Inflammation serves a vital function in the human body, as it communicates problems and may aid in healing, such as when the inflammation of a sprained ankle forces the sufferer to rest the injured ankle. When inflammation exists for a prolonged period, though, it becomes a risk, as it negatively impacts cellular function. The relation of inflammation to many diseases of the body is recognized, but its connection to brain disease is not known by the public, possibly because people can't feel inflammation in the brain the way they can when it manifests in joints in the form of arthritis. Anti-inflammatories and antioxidants, such as Vitamins A, C, and E, help reduce inflammation and lower risk of neurological illness. Exercise and sleep also play a role in neurological health and controlling inflammation.

Statins, prescribed to combat high cholesterol, are touted as anti-inflammatory, but studies show that they may negatively impact brain function and contribute to heart disease. Neurons rely on the fuel they receive from cholesterol; without it, they cease to function properly.

Key Take-Aways

- Accepted teachings that a diet high in carbohydrates and low in fat is healthy are wrong. Humans evolved to require a diet rich in healthy fat and low in carbohydrates.

- Cholesterol is vital to the brain's health.

CHAPTER 2

Summary

A number of dissimilar case histories, such as chronic migraines, severe mood issues (depression), and movement disorders (involuntary twitching and muscle spasms), have been proven to be alleviated by adhering to a gluten-free diet. Gluten is a protein that holds flour together in bread products, and it is present in a variety of grains. It's found in products ranging from bread to personal hygiene items and even cheese.

The stickiness of gluten interferes with the body's ability to break down nutrients. The residue of undigested food sets off a reaction that culminates in inflammation that may increase the risk of autoimmune disease. The resultant chemicals, cytokines, are found in a number of brain diseases.

Though considered a modern ailment, celiac disease was noted in first century AD Greek writings and found in numerous studies throughout history, though its cause was unknown until the 1940s. The link between celiac disease and neurological disorders was first noted in the 1800s and continued to be documented through the 1900s. However, the assumption was that the neurological disorders were considered manifestations of the celiac disease. Not until 2005 did doctors consider gluten's effect on the brain, due to a greater understanding of inflammation. Gluten sensitivity is not confined to the gut; it always affects the brain. It's possible that everyone is sensitive to gluten neurologically, even if they don't show evidence of it, due to its inflammatory properties.

Due to hybridization, today's wheat is radically different from the wheat human ancestors first ate. Whereas gluten has changed genetically, the people eating it have not undergone the same level of change.

Consumption of gluten causes a hormonal reaction in the body that mimics the effects of opiates, imparting feelings of euphoria. Food manufacturers know this and pack their foods with gluten.

The glycemic index measures how rapidly blood sugar rises in response to food. Between the choices of a tablespoon of sugar, a candy bar, a banana, and a slice of whole wheat bread, the item with

the highest glycemic index is the slice of
bread.

Key Take-Aways

- Gluten sensitivity manifests in areas
other than the bowels and causes
inflammation throughout the body,
including the brain.

- The human diet has changed from
what humans evolved to require.

CHAPTER 3

Summary

Gluten isn't the only villain attacking the brain's health; all carbohydrates are bad. A diet high in fat (not from processed foods) and low in carbohydrates is what humans have evolved to need and on which they thrive. Foods high in fat do not cause obesity; foods high in cholesterol do not cause high cholesterol; and high cholesterol does not increase cardiac risk.

Humans evolved a "thrifty gene" to help them store fat to sustain them through times of famine. That gene remains and is linked to obesity and type 2 diabetes.

Autopsies of the brains of Alzheimer's patients display significantly lower fat content and cholesterol levels than are found in a healthy brain, regardless of whether the patient was genetically predisposed to Alzheimer's disease. Further studies indicate people who regularly consume fish and oils rich in omega-3 fats are significantly less likely to develop neurological diseases. People who regularly consume the more common omega-6 oils double their risk of dementia. Studies also show that people with lower levels of cholesterol are at greater risk of dementia, memory loss, and Parkinson's disease. Problems only arise with cholesterol when carbohydrates interfere, impeding its function of carrying nutrients to the brain. Studies of patients with low and high cholesterol showed no difference in their rates of heart attack and mortality. Further, studies of hundreds of thousands of subjects have shown there is no correlation between saturated fat and increased risk for "coronary heart disease, stroke, or cardiovascular disease." In fact, risk was lowest in people consuming the highest level of saturated fat.

The surge in blood sugar that follows consumption of carbohydrates has a domino effect on the body. It depletes a number of neurotransmitters (which regulates mood and brain), burns through vital B-complex vitamins, diminishes magnesium levels, and increases glycation (the combination of glucose, proteins, and fats). Glycation in particular contributes to brain tissue shrinkage. When the American government recommended a high-carb diet in 1992, and the American Diabetes Association followed suit, the rate of diabetes soared, doubling between 1997 and 2007.

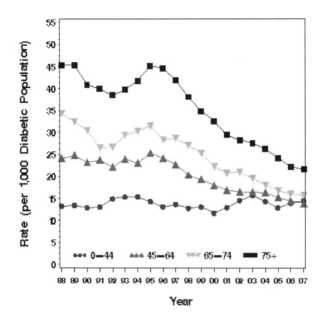

(Image courtesy of cdc.gov)

Good fat is vital to a healthy body. It reduces inflammation and allows vitamin absorption. This includes saturated fats, which every cell in the body needs. Fat is the "superfuel" of the brain, which is made up of 70 percent fat. The brain contains 25 percent of the body's total cholesterol. Cholesterol allows the brain to communicate and function properly, and it works as an antioxidant. A diet rich in healthy fats and cholesterol has been demonized, and one benefactor is Big Pharma and the billions it makes pushing statins on the public. Statins have numerous side effects, including memory lapses, confusion, and a dramatic increase in diabetes risk. Statins negatively impact the liver's cholesterol-making abilities, promoting neurological disorders. There are also a number of detrimental side effects that increase risk for a large number of ailments and diseases, as well as little evidence that they work for their intended purpose, other than the fact they do work as an anti-inflammatory. Additionally, research reveals a link between statins and increased cancer risk. The body creates cholesterol, far more than is consumed through diet, and cutting cholesterol causes the body to create it from excess carbohydrates and store it, as when in famine mode. This cycle of overproduction continues, causing high cholesterol. Patients who undergo a high cholesterol diet see their cholesterol levels drop without drug interaction.

Key Take-Aways

- Fat is necessary to fuel the brain and keep it functioning correctly.

- Cholesterol is good for the body and the brain; a diet low in cholesterol is devastating for the body on many levels.

- There is no correlation between high cholesterol and heart disease.

CHAPTER 4

Summary

Excess sugar, especially refined or processed sugar, has been proven detrimental to the body. Fructose is the sugar that occurs naturally in fruit and honey. Glucose is the sugar created from carbohydrates. Sucrose, or table sugar, is a combination of glucose and fructose. High-fructose corn syrup is found in many processed foods and drinks and receives the bulk of the blame for obesity and other health problems. In reality, all sugars and carbohydrates (which are made of sugar molecules) are the cause of these health issues. Increased carbohydrates, specifically glucose, cause the pancreas to increase insulin output. Due to this, carbs that increase blood sugar the most are also the ones that are most fattening.

The carbohydrates found in vegetables are combined with fiber, so they break down slower and don't have the same kind of impact on the bloodstream. The sugars in whole fruits also have less impact than starchy carbs, though they have a greater impact than vegetables. Fruit juices, even those that are 100 percent from fruit, have the same impact as soda, though, because the fiber has been removed and the sugar immediately hits the bloodstream. The liver converts these sugars to fat cells, and over time, may cause insulin resistance and increase fat storage.

To guard against diabetes, balancing blood sugar is key. Numerous studies show that diabetes is associated with decreased cognitive function and increased risk of brain diseases. The earlier a person is diagnosed with diabetes, the greater the risk and severity of cognitive decline.

Proteins form the basic structure of the entire body, and deformed proteins are found in all neurological disorders. These proteins have the ability to infect surrounding healthy cells, and the damage is irreversible. Glycation (bonded sugar, protein, fat, and amino acids) causes these proteins to become deformed. Glycation is inevitable, but it can be retarded by adhering to a low-carb diet.

Hemoglobin A1C is a glycated protein that doctors test to gauge blood sugar. Elevated hemoglobin A1C indicates risk for diabetes, stroke, heart disease, and brain atrophy. Reduced carbs and increased exercise lower hemoglobin A1C counts.

Excess weight carries significant

danger. Visceral fat envelopes vital organs and triggers inflammation; it is linked to an enormous number of health problems, including brain dysfunction. Visceral fat is unseen, but waist size is a good indicator of its severity. Studies show that the larger a person's waist, the smaller the hippocampus (the brain's memory center). Additionally, risk for stroke and dementia increases with waist size. Studies prove that exercise alone does not improve insulin and blood sugar levels; a low-carb, high-fat diet must also be incorporated. This diet also shows the most long-term success, with individuals more likely to maintain the healthier weight.

Key Take-Aways

- Sugars are the most fattening and dangerous substance for the body, and carbohydrates are comprised of strings of sugar molecules.

- Deformed proteins are the basis of disease, including brain ailments, and they infect surrounding cells.

- Obesity is directly related to brain size and function: the bigger the body, the smaller the brain. Low-carb, high-fat diets are best for reducing weight.

CHAPTER 5

Summary

People can reprogram their DNA to return to optimum health. Epigenetics studies the "marks" that determine how genes express themselves. Lifestyle affects these marks; over 70 percent of the genes related to health and longevity can be manipulated through lifestyle choices.

The idea that brain neurons do not regenerate has been disproved. Brain-derived neurotrophic factor (BDNF) protects existing neurons and helps create new ones. Alzheimer's patients have decreased BDNF levels. Exercise and proper diet positively influence BDNF production. Physical exercise is a powerful method of genetic change. Aerobic exercise activates genes connected to longevity and targets the brain's growth hormone. Reduced calorie diets also increase BDNF production, and studies show improved memory and mental faculties. These same benefits can be gained by consuming fats known as ketones. One of the most important brain "fats" is docosahexaenoic acid (DHA), which makes up one-quarter of the brain's weight. DHA supplements have been proven to increase memory, lower risk for Alzheimer's and dementia, and treat disorders like ADHD. Studies show it also, along with other omega-3 fats, dramatically reduces free radicals.

Stimulating the brain intellectually is also vital to its health and the production of neurons. The brain's speed and efficiency increase, as does its capacity. People who meditate also lower their risk of brain disease.

No gene causes Alzheimer's, but there is a genetic risk factor called the ApoE Ɛ4 allele, which is found in approximately 25 percent of the population and 40 percent of Alzheimer's patients. The presence of this marker does not guarantee a person will contract Alzheimer's disease; it only presents an increased risk. Lifestyle changes can lower this risk.

Key Take-Aways

- It is possible to reprogram genes through diet and exercise.

- Lifestyle changes dramatically reduce risk for brain diseases and increase neural growth, even for individuals with a genetic predisposition to Alzheimer's.

CHAPTER 6

Summary

In addition to lowering risk for Alzheimer's and dementia, a gluten-free diet effects radical changes in behaviors associated with ADHD without resorting to drug therapy. Incidence of children being diagnosed with ADHD has increased rapidly in recent years, and their doctors regularly prescribe mind-altering drugs to combat the disorder. ADHD diagnoses rose 53 percent in the past decade. Also on the rise are prescriptions for anti-anxiety medications: 45 percent in females and 37 percent in males. In general, prescriptions to address mental health issues have increased; one in five Americans takes one of these drugs. Little attention has been paid to the source of these mental health issues. Could gluten sensitivity be the root cause? Scientists do know celiac disease may increase risk of neurological disorders. Additionally, gluten-sensitive patients suffer depression and anxiety due to blockage of neurotransmitters. Studies and case histories of individuals with ADHD and other brain disorders reveal dramatic improvement of symptoms with the removal of gluten, without using drug therapy.

Depression is commonly treated with drug therapy. Antidepressant drugs have severe side effects, both mental and physical in nature. For patients with mild forms of depression, alternative therapies may prove more beneficial. Studies prove depression and suicide risk is higher in people with low cholesterol, including those who take statins. Celiac patients and those with gluten sensitivity also have a much higher risk of depression and suicide. This is due to the gut's inability to absorb nutrients once it's been injured by celiac disease. These nutrients are necessary for the production of neurological chemicals. Additionally, many "feel-good" hormones are produced in nerve cells near the intestines, including approximately 85 percent of the body's serotonin. Many patients for whom antidepressants don't work find relief by adopting a gluten-free diet. When treating any of these disorders, time must be allowed for the changes to take effect, usually 90 days at minimum.

Many issues are at play for mental illnesses such as schizophrenia and bipolar disorder, but often people with these diagnoses display gluten sensitivity. A history of celiac disease also significantly increases risk for these disorders. Children born to gluten-sensitive mothers have a 50 percent higher risk of developing schizophrenia later in life. Case histories of patients with schizophrenia and histories of hallucinations, depression, and suicide attempts have shown reversal of symptoms by removing gluten from their diet.

Chronic headaches may also be relieved by a gluten-free diet. Migraine sufferers are also more likely to suffer from celiac disease or gluten sensitivity. The inflammation associated with gluten consumption may be to blame. Many of the drugs used to treat headaches come with alarming side effects, especially for children. Waist size is also a good predictor of headaches, including migraines. Studies show that excess belly fat significantly increases migraine activity and chronic headaches. Healthy lifestyle choices can cure headaches permanently.

Key Take-Aways

- Eliminating gluten activates the body's natural healing capabilities and offers relief for behavioral disorders and possibly mental illness.

- Low-carb, high-cholesterol diets combined with exercise will cure chronic headaches and migraines without drug intervention.

CHAPTER 7

Summary

The size of the human brain as a percentage of total body weight dwarfs the rest of the animal kingdom: 1/40. The amount of energy the brain consumes is even greater: 22 percent of the body's at-rest energy expenditure.

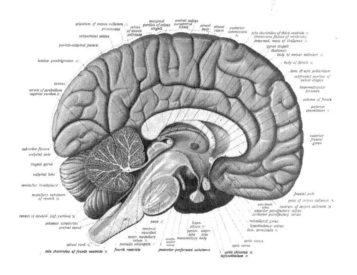

(Photo courtesy of Wikipedia.org)

Intermittent fasting, not eating for 24 to 72 hours, nourishes the brain. Beta-hydroxybutyrate (beta-HBA) is the brain's principal ketone, a super fuel that produces energy efficiently and protects neurons. Beta-HBA comes into play after about three days of fasting. Its benefits to the brain are substantial and can be added to the diet through coconut oil. Fasting accelerates and enhances weight loss and increases brain health. It increases BDNF production, enhances detoxification, reduces inflammation, and causes the brain to use fat for fuel instead of glucose.

A ketogenic diet mimics the diet of caveman days, and its calories are approximately 85 percent fat-based, with the remainder coming from carbohydrates and protein. Ketones are far more effective than glucose as brain fuel.

Supplements help focus on prevention of illness rather than treatment.

1. DHA is an omega-3 fatty acid that comprises over 90 percent of the brain's fats. It can be found in supplement form or in enhanced food products.

2. Resveratrol is a natural compound that slows aging, increases blood flow to the brain, and Improves heart health. It is found in grapes and red wine. One glass of red wine a day is a health benefit, but supplements are needed for the higher doses required to obtain resveratrol's many benefits.

3. Turmeric is a member of the ginger family with remarkable anti-inflammatory and antioxidant properties.

4. Probiotics influence brain behavior and alleviate stress, anxiety, and depression.

5. Coconut oil helps prevent and treat neurodegenerative disease states; it is a super fuel for the brain and an anti-inflammatory.

6. Alpha-lipoic acid is a fatty acid found in each cell of the body, where it produces energy and acts as an antioxidant.

7. Vitamin D is a steroid hormone with receptors throughout the nervous system. Reduced levels dramatically increase risk for a wide range of neurological disorders and diseases.

Key Take-Aways

- Maintaining a low ketotic state is beneficial on many levels. This state can be obtained by adhering to a ketogenic diet.

- Intermittent fasting has many benefits.

- Supplements are necessary for optimum health.

CHAPTER 8

Summary

Exercise is key to brain health. Aerobic exercise makes people smarter, activates longevity genes, and targets BDNF, the brain's growth hormone. It may also reverse memory decline. Alzheimer's risk increases as exercise levels decrease. Human genes require aerobic exercise to sustain life. Studies prove the link between exercise and improved cognitive thinking, and aerobic exercise is the winner over other forms of activity. Higher levels of BDNF also decrease appetite, another benefit of exercise. Regular exercise improves insulin sensitivity, helps manage blood sugar, and reduces glycation.

The level of exercise intensity has a direct impact on risk for brain disease, but all levels of physical activity help alleviate risk. Running displays the best results, but 20 minutes per day, five days per week of any aerobic activity shows similar benefits.

Key Take-Aways

- Human brains evolved to their current size thanks to the aerobic exercise of the hunter-gatherer lifestyle.

- The human body requires aerobic exercise to maintain health.

- Aerobic exercise greatly improves brain health.

CHAPTER 9

Summary

Sleep is essential to well-being and building a healthy brain. It dictates how people eat, metabolism, weight, ability to fight disease, cognitive powers, and ability to cope with stress. Adequate sleep also affects genes. Quantity of sleep is not the only measure of adequate sleep; quality also counts. People with disrupted sleep, such as sleep apnea, have more than double the risk of dementia in their later years.

Circadian rhythms are developed by the age of six weeks and affect sleep cycles, hormones, and body temperature. Shift workers, with their irregular sleep patterns, have higher risk for a number of illnesses. Uncharacteristic changes in mood or attitude may be explained by examining recent sleep habits.

Leptin is a hormone that influences all other hormones and controls most of the functions of the hypothalamus, which is "responsible for the body's rhythmic activities and physiological functions." Leptin is found in fat cells and is a basic survival tool, with powerful influence on feelings and behaviors. Understanding leptin will allow a person to manage his or her health, as it controls the thyroid and therefore metabolism. Fat cells release leptin to announce that the stomach is full. If leptin levels are low, people overeat, and sleep deprivation causes leptin levels to plunge. Leptin also controls inflammation in the body and is negatively affected by carbohydrates. An overabundance of leptins, which is triggered by excessive carb consumption, causes leptin resistance, so the brain ignores its messages. There is no supplement or drug to control leptin; it can only be controlled by adequate sleep and smart dietary choices.

Ghrelin is another appetite-related hormone, secreted by the stomach to indicate hunger. Sleep deprivation causes ghrelin levels to soar at the same time leptin levels plummet. The brain becomes disconnected from the stomach, and cravings for comfort food are hard to resist, perpetuating the cycle.

Key Take-Aways

- Sleep is vital to overall health, both in quantity and quality.

- Hormones that control appetite and hunger are negatively affected by poor sleep habits, leading to obesity and a host of ailments, including neurological disorders.

CHAPTER 10

Summary

Readers may be apprehensive about their ability to cut carbs from their diets and maintain this new lifestyle. Adhering to this four-week plan, though, will provide the kind of results that inspire belief and dedication in these changes. Before beginning, check with a physician, especially if you have preexisting conditions, such as diabetes. The goals of the next four weeks:

1. Shift away from carbs and add daily supplements

2. Incorporate fitness

3. Get restful sleep

4. Establish and maintain healthy habits

Before beginning, prepare by having the following tests performed:

1. Fasting blood glucose

2. Fasting insulin

3. Hemoglobin A1C

4. Fructosamine

5. Homocysteine

6. Vitamin D

7. C-reactive protein

8. Gluten sensitivity with Cyrex array 3 test

Repeat these tests upon completion of the four weeks. It may take several months to see dramatic changes, but some improvement should be evident after the initial four weeks. Additionally, use this preparation time to begin daily supplements. Refer to your doctor for specific dosages, or follow the recommendations below:

1. Alpha lipoic acid: 600 mg daily

2. Coconut oil: 1 teaspoon orally or use in cooking

3. DHA: 1,000 mg daily (DHA combined with EPA is fine)

4. Probiotics: 1 capsule on an empty stomach, up to three times/day

5. Resveratrol: 100 mg twice daily

6. Turmeric: 350 mg twice daily

7. Vitamin D3: 5,000 IU daily

Prepare your kitchen, as well, by removing the following:

1. All sources of gluten

2. All forms of processed carbs, sugar, and starch

3. Packaged foods labeled "fat free" or "low fat"

4. Margarine and vegetable shortening or oil

5. Non-fermented soy and processed foods made with soy

6. Avoid foods labeled "gluten-free"

Add the following items, using organic and local wherever possible:

1. Healthy fat

2. Herbs, seasonings, and condiments

3. Low-sugar fruit

4. Protein

5. Vegetables

To be used in moderation:

1. Carrots and parsnips

2. Cottage cheese, yogurt, kefir

3. Cow's milk and cream

4. Legumes (except chickpeas)

5. Non-gluten grains

6. Sweeteners

7. Whole sweet fruit

8. Wine (one glass/day)

The ideal way to start week one is after fasting for 24 hours; no food, but plenty of water and avoid caffeine, and continue taking medications. If unable or unwilling to fast, wean yourself off carbs for a few days, and cut all gluten.

Week one focuses on food. There is no calorie counting or worry about fats. The meals will leave you feeling full for hours, eliminate cravings, and prevent afternoon brain fog. This first month differs from the lifetime plan in that carbs are lower, only 30 to 40 grams daily. After, items from the "moderate" category may be added. A food journal may be helpful as you learn which foods you like. Avoid eating out the first few weeks while you learn the ropes.

Week two focuses on exercise, with the goal of 20 minutes daily of aerobic activity as a minimum. These are habits for a lifetime, so don't push too hard, too fast, but do challenge yourself. If you already maintain a fitness regimen, try to increase to a minimum of 30 minutes per day, five times per week. Eventually, your workout will include cardio, strength, and stretch training, but begin with cardio. In addition, change your routine occasionally, try new things, and schedule time to exercise. If there are days that truly offer no time to exercise for an extended period, look for ways to sneak in physical activity. Three 10-minute bouts offer the same benefits as one 30-minute session. Find ways to incorporate more movement into your daily life.

Week three focuses on sleep. Sleep should have improved by following the protocols for two weeks; the goal is seven hours per night minimum. Some tips for a good night's sleep:

1. Maintain regular sleep habits: go to bed and wake at roughly the same time every day

2. Identify and manage ingredients hostile to sleep: caffeine, alcohol, nicotine (adopt a plan to quit smoking)

3. Time dinner appropriately: approximately three hours before bedtime

4. Don't eat erratically: eat on a schedule

5. Try a bedtime snack: foods high in tryptophan, being careful of portion size

6. Beware of stimulants: caffeine and other stimulants hide everywhere

7. Set the setting: limited electronics, dim lighting, comfortable bedding

8. Use sleep aids prudently

Go through toiletries now to remove

products with gluten, such as lotions, shampoos, and body washes (to name only a few) and replace with gluten-free products.

Week four puts all of this together. At this point, you should feel better, understand the healthier food choices, enjoy improved sleep, and exercise routinely. Identify areas of struggle and look for solutions. Pointers:

1. Plan each week in advance

2. Prepare shopping lists

3. Create "non-negotiable" goals

4. Use technology

5. Be flexible but consistent

6. Find motivators

A goal for the end of week four is to eat out while staying on plan. Once established in this new lifestyle, the occasional splurge, like a slice of pizza, will occur, but don't let it become the norm. Try a 90/10 rule: eat within these guidelines 90 percent of the time, splurge 10 percent. If you fall off the wagon, fast for a day and restart the four weeks of 30 to 40 carbs per day.

Key Take-Aways

- Prepare before beginning this new plan.

- Week one focuses on food.

- Week two focuses on exercise.

- Week three focuses on sleep.

- Week four brings it all together.

CHAPTER 11

Summary

These recipes prove the choices for this lifestyle are plentiful, and they provide a jumping off point for planning your own menus. They require no calorie, protein, or fat counting, and you won't feel underfed. Choose organic or wild foods whenever possible, and choose produce in season.

Drink half your bodyweight in ounces of purified water daily, i.e., 150 pounds equals 75 ounces of water. You may add tea or coffee, being careful of caffeinated drinks later in the day. Add 12 to 16 ounces of water for every caffeinated beverage. A glass of wine, preferably red, is permitted with dinner.

Whole fruit during the first four weeks should be eaten as a snack or dessert. Olive oil may be used liberally for cooking, or coconut oil may be substituted. Precook foods like chicken and beef to bring for lunch or have on hand in your refrigerator. Prepare greens and chopped vegetables for quick salad, adding protein and dressing immediately before eating. Canned foods like salmon and tomatoes are helpful; just read labels for ingredients like sugar.

Snacking is permitted. Suggestions: raw nuts (except peanuts), olives, dark chocolate, raw vegetables (dipped in hummus, guacamole, goat cheese, tapenade, or cheese and wheat-free nut butter), low-carb crackers, sliced poultry, half an avocado, two hard-boiled eggs, Caprese salad, cold (and peeled) shrimp, and one serving whole, low-sugar fruit. The recipes included are simple to prepare, taste delicious, and make following the plan for the first week simple.

Key Take-Aways

- High-fat, low-carb foods are delicious and satisfying.

- Follow the suggested menu and food choices to make integrating this new lifestyle easy.

EPILOGUE

Summary

People are subjected to brilliantly marketed health claims daily and bombarded with conflicting messages about health; it's hard to know what's true. Not long ago, people were told eggs are terrible and margarine is healthy; now, the opposite is known to be true. Sixty years ago, doctors advertised for cigarettes. Sixty years from now, what current doctor-professed "good" will be debunked?

America spends nearly 20 percent of its GDP on healthcare. It is ranked first in healthcare expenditures but 37th in overall health-system performance and 22nd in life expectancy. To save ourselves and future generations, we must make individual changes in lifestyle.

The brain is the center of human health, and it can be nurtured by following the changes prescribed.

Key Take-Aways

- Don't believe claims of what's healthy and what isn't; throughout history, the medical community has been wrong.

- Take control of your health.

PUTTING IT TOGETHER

Grain Brain makes the case that diet influences brain health the same way it affects body health. Since the 1990s, diabetes rates have soared in America, as have various mental and behavioral disorders. People with diabetes are twice as likely to develop Alzheimer's disease. All of these, though, are preventable with lifestyle changes: cut gluten, reduce carbs, increase healthy fats, exercise more, and get plenty of sleep.

Dr. Perlmutter answers the question of how to effectively improve health through diet and exercise, and he offers an easy-to-follow plan to implement his recommended lifestyle changes. The menu, diet choices, and recipes he includes are added bonuses and offer a simple way to begin. What he doesn't address is how expensive it would be to implement this diet. Grass-fed and free-range meats are significantly more expensive than commonly found items at the local grocer. Additionally, the fresh produce and herbs he recommends readers fill their plates with also come with a much higher price tag than potatoes, pasta, and rice.

Perlmutter presents his scientific evidence with levels of knowledge and confidence that are convincing, but which deflate somewhat upon research. Reviews of *Grain Brain* often include interviews with doctors and scientists refuting his theories. To support his claims, he presents faulty historical evidence of diet and health. Perlmutter also ignores the current eating habits of different cultures that follow a high-carb diet with low or non-existent levels of brain disease.

His arguments that doctors too-readily treat disease and neurological ailments with drug therapy are convincing. The surge in prescriptions to treat disorders like ADHD and depression are troubling, as long-term effects of these drugs are unknown. If changes to diet can affect change without the use of mind-altering drugs, especially in children, that will be a very positive outcome of his research.

ABOUT THE BOOK'S AUTHOR

Dr. David Perlmutter is a neurologist whose medical practice is in Naples, Florida. He is also a Fellow of the American College of Nutrition. He received his M.D. from the University of Miami School of Medicine, where he was awarded the Leonard G. Rowntree Research Award and now serves as an Associate Professor.

Dr. Perlmutter is a frequent lecturer at leading universities, and he is a well-known proponent of using a holistic approach to not only treat but also prevent neurological dysfunction. He has received a number of awards for his work in treating and preventing brain diseases. In 2002, he was given both the Linus Pauling Award and Denham Harman Award. He is the 2006 recipient of the National Nutritional Foods Association Clinician of the Year. In 2010, the American College of Nutrition named him Humanitarian of the Year.

Prior to *Grain Brain*, David Perlmutter published three books: *Power Up Your Brain: The Neuroscience of Enlightenment*, *The Better Brain Book: The Best Tool for Improving Memory and Sharpness and Preventing Aging of the Brain*, and *Raise a*

Smarter Child by Kindergarten. In addition to his published books, Dr. Perlmutter contributes extensively to medical publications worldwide. He is also a frequent contributor to popular publications such as *Huffington Post*.

Perlmutter is a frequent guest on a number of news programs, talk shows, and 24-hour news networks. He also serves as a medical advisor for *The Doctor Oz Show*. He considers himself an "empowering neurologist," and his goal is to help people take control of their diet, their genes, and their health, by sharing the facts of what he considers the brain's silent killers: gluten and carbohydrates.

To learn more about Dr. Perlmutter and *Grain Brain*, visit his website: www.drperlmutter.com.

Readers Who Enjoyed This Ebook Might Also Enjoy...

Dr. David Perlmutter's _Grain Brain: The Surprising Truth about Wheat, Carbs, and Sugar--Your Brain's Silent Killers_ (the full book)

Dr. Terry Wahl's _The Wahls Protocol_

Jane Olson's _Counting Calories_

Save Time Summaries' _Summary of Fat Chance -- Battling Sugar, Obesity & Disease by Robert Lustig_

#

30944588R00038

Made in the USA
Lexington, KY
24 March 2014